Ines Naceur

Niemann-Pick type B disease in adulthood: a diagnostic challenge

Ines Naceur

Niemann-Pick type B disease in adulthood: a diagnostic challenge

ScienciaScripts

Imprint

Any brand names and product names mentioned in this book are subject to trademark, brand or patent protection and are trademarks or registered trademarks of their respective holders. The use of brand names, product names, common names, trade names, product descriptions etc. even without a particular marking in this work is in no way to be construed to mean that such names may be regarded as unrestricted in respect of trademark and brand protection legislation and could thus be used by anyone.

Cover image: www.ingimage.com

This book is a translation from the original published under ISBN 978-620-6-72361-5.

Publisher:
Sciencia Scripts
is a trademark of
Dodo Books Indian Ocean Ltd. and OmniScriptum S.R.L publishing group

120 High Road, East Finchley, London, N2 9ED, United Kingdom
Str. Armeneasca 28/1, office 1, Chisinau MD-2012, Republic of Moldova, Europe
Printed at: see last page
ISBN: 978-620-8-16110-1

NIEMANN-PICK TYPE B DISEASE IN OLD AGE ADULTS: A DIAGNOSTIC CHALLENGE

DR INES NACEUR

I dedicate this work to all my loved ones: my family, my friends and my colleagues...

PLAN

INTRODUCTION 7

CHAPTER 1.. 11

CHAPTER 2.. 19

CHAPTER 3.. 22

CHAPTER 4.. 27

CHAPTER 5.. 29

CHAPTER 6.. 31

CHAPTER 7.. 33

CONCLUSIONS 36

REFERENCES 38

ABSTRACT

Niemann-Pick disease type B (NP-B) or acid sphingomyelinase deficiency (DSMA) is an autosomal recessive lysosomal storage disease caused by a mutation in the sphingomyelin phosphodiesterase 1 (SMPD1) gene. SMPD is responsible for an accumulation of sphingomyelin in lysosomes and abnormalities in the lipid constituents of cell membranes.

Clinically, there are three entities secondary to DSMA: Niemann-Pick type A disease (NP-A), which is an early neurovisceral form; Niemann-Pick type B disease, which is a chronic visceral form; and Niemann-Pick type A/B disease (NP-A/B), which is a chronic neurovisceral form. NP-A disease is characterised by severe visceral and neurodegenerative damage that is progressive and fatal within the first three years of life. In B forms, there is no neurological involvement and the age of onset is highly variable, with adult onset possible.

The clinical picture often combines almost constant hepatosplenomegaly, interstitial lung disease (usually asymptomatic or manifested by recurrent pulmonary infections), joint pain, diarrhoea and delayed growth and puberty.

The course of the disease is fairly heterogeneous, with variable phenotypes and intermediate forms have been described.

The heterogeneity of systemic manifestations and the sometimes late onset of the disease are the main reasons for misdiagnosis in adulthood.

INTRODUCTION

Lysosomal storage disorders (LSDs) account for a large number (>50) of hereditary metabolic disorders (IMDs). These rare or even exceptional diseases are linked to a disturbance in the catabolism of complex molecules, which gradually accumulate in various tissues (1). The biochemical anomalies responsible may be a deficiency of a lysosomal enzyme, a deficiency of the activator protein or a cofactor of a lysosomal enzyme, a deficiency of a protein that stabilises a lysosomal enzyme complex, a defect in the extra-lysosomal maturation of the enzyme or a deficiency of a lysosomal membrane transporter (2). Acid sphingomyelinase deficiency (ASMD) or Niemann-Pick disease (NP) is a disease of lysosomal overload, secondary as its name suggests to an enzyme deficiency in acid sphingomyelinase (ASM) (3). It is an autosomal recessive disease. There are three forms of DSMA: the infantile neurovisceral form or Niemann-Pick type A disease (NP-A), the chronic visceral form or Niemann-Pick type B disease (NP-B), and the chronic neurovisceral form or Niemann-Pick type A/B disease (NP- A/B). Niemann-Pick type C disease, which is due to an abnormality in intracellular lipid trafficking, is therefore not included in the DSMA group. NP-A disease is the rarest and most severe form, with an incidence of less than 1/10,000 and severe neurovegetative and visceral manifestations. This form often manifests itself in early childhood, with a fatal course in the first three years of life (4).

NP-B or DSMA-B disease is a chronic visceral form, more common than type A, affecting around one in 500,000 people, and is often less severe (5,6).

Symptoms vary: pulmonary, hepatic, splenic, digestive, articular and bony, with no neurological involvement except in intermediate forms A/B (chronic neurovisceral form) (3,6). Pulmonary involvement is often asymptomatic and may be revealed by pulmonary infections, dyspnoea or crackles on auscultation (7,8).

The most common sign is hepatosplenomegaly, with a risk of progression of liver damage to hepatocellular failure and cirrhosis (9). Liver failure and respiratory failure are the two main causes of death in this disease (10). The age of onset varies widely. Generally diagnosed in childhood, it may be discovered in adulthood (1114).

Diagnostic confirmation is initially achieved by measuring SMA enzyme activity, the residual level of which does not confirm the type. Genetic testing for a mutation in the SMPD1 gene is the reference method for diagnostic confirmation (15).

The variability of the clinical presentation and the late age of onset of the disease often raise the problem of differential diagnosis with infectious or inflammatory systemic diseases or with other MHMs.

CHAPTER 1

ACID SPHINGOMYELINASE DEFICIENCY IN ADULTHOOD:

FROM MECHANISM TO MANIFESTATIONS CLINICS

1. Liver damage

Hepatomegaly is one of the most frequent manifestations of DSMA-B and is seen in up to 70% of cases of Niemann-Pick type B disease. Liver volume is often correlated with hypersplenism and the severity of extrahepatic manifestations (16).

Hepatomegaly is secondary to the accumulation of sphingomyelin in hepatocytes and Kupffer cells. Increases in aspartate aminotransferase (ASAT), alanine aminotransferase (ALAT) and total bilirubin are common but do not appear to correlate with the stage of fibrosis or the severity of liver damage (6). The course is variable, with possible progression to cirrhosis and hepatocellular failure (6,10-12). In a systematic analysis of liver biopsies taken from adult patients with type B DSMA, hepatic fibrosis was observed in 88% of patients (12). Some of these patients had frank cirrhosis in the absence of any clinical symptoms of liver failure. The 17 reference biopsies showed variable levels of accumulated SMA (12).

Patients homozygous for the SMPD1 gene mutation, which is often associated with moderate to severe forms of the disease, have a higher incidence of liver damage, with more frequent progression to cirrhosis (17). Hepatocellular failure is one of the main causes of mortality in the course of the disease. Progression to hepatocellular carcinoma is possible but rare (5,9,10,18).

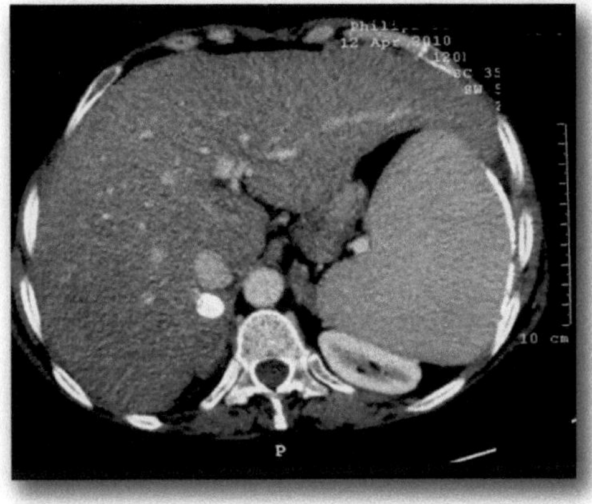

Figure 1: Abdominal section showing hepatomegaly and hepatic calcifications in a 51-year-old patient with type B acid sphingomyelinase deficiency.

2. Splenic involvement

Splenomegaly is one of the most frequent manifestations of DSMA and is often the first obvious sign of the disease. It may be asymptomatic, discovered by chance, or massive and symptomatic, with abdominal pain, feelings of abdominal discomfort and early satiety. Splenomegaly can be massive and is often correlated with the severity of the disease. Hypersplenism may be complicated by infarction and secondary cytopenias (6,18,19).

3. Lung disease

This mode of revelation is considered unusual in adults, as diffuse infiltrative lung disease is often asymptomatic and rarely reveals the disease (13,20). Pulmonary involvement may be asymptomatic, discovered by chance, or may manifest as recurrent pulmonary infections or variable dyspnoea. Severe forms with respiratory failure may also be seen (7,8,20-22).

Lung damage progresses slowly but inevitably due to the progressive accumulation of Niemann-Pick cells in the alveolar septa, bronchial walls and pleura, which explains the restrictive ventilatory disorders reported (8). Bronchoalveolar lavage is of diagnostic value, revealing multivacuolate histiocytes containing fine and coarse granules that stain deep blue with the May-

Grunwald-Giemsa stain, known as "sea-blue histiocytes" or Niemann-Pick cells (23). Thoracic computed tomographyoften shows ground-glass areas and thickening of the interlobular and intralobular septa, giving a "crazy paving" appearance (23,24). Lung infiltration explains the abnormalities reported on functional tests. Carbon monoxide diffusion capacity (DLCO) may be reduced even if lung volume is normal (25). Lung biopsy and/or BAL may reveal features of lipoid pneumonia, including infiltration by Niemann-Pick cells (25).

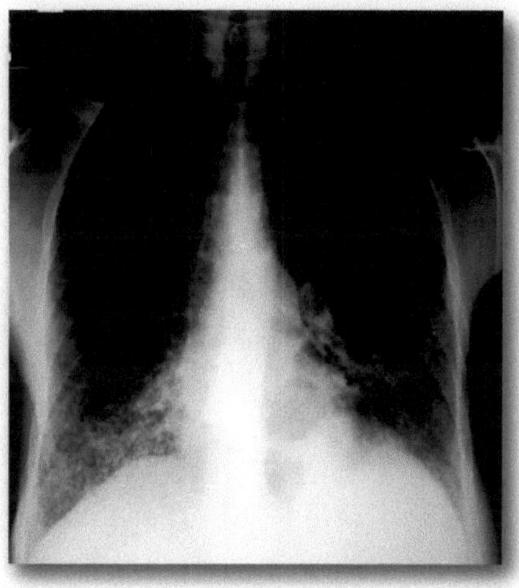

Figure 2: Chest X-ray showing interstitial syndrome in a 51-year-old patient with type B acid sphingomyelinase deficiency.

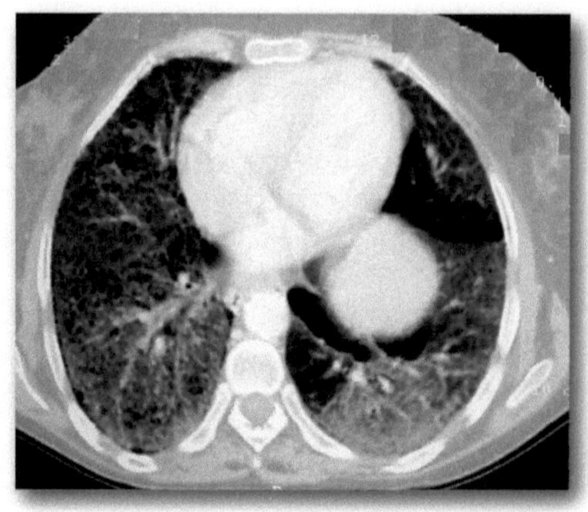

Figure 3: Chest CT scan showing diffuse interstitial lung disease

in a 51-year-old patient with type B acid sphingomyelinase

deficiency.

4. Adrenal damage

Adrenal involvement has been reported in a few cases in the

literature. This was reported in the study of three familial cases

published by C. Alizon et al (26). These three patients had

multiple punctiform parenchymal calcifications giving a "starry

sky" appearance, as well as bilateral adrenal hyperplasia (26).

5. Eye damage

Ocular involvement is common in Niemann-Pick type B disease, manifested by a cherry-red patch in the macula (16).

6. Musculoskeletal damage

Skeletal involvement is also common and includes osteopenia, osteoporosis, bone pain and fractures (27). Bone density abnormalities may affect one or more sites (27). This condition is often complicated by delayed development and growth (6,16). However, adult height may be normal or at the lower limit of normal (6).

The pathophysiology of skeletal damage in DSMA is not well understood. well understood. The use of bisphosphonate in DSMA is controversial. This molecule may inhibit the activity of acid sphingomyelinase and therefore risk aggravating the disease (27,28).

7. Haematological disorders

Haematological abnormalities are inconstant in DSMA type B. These abnormalities vary in severity. Thrombocytopenia is the most common haematological abnormality and is often moderate. Leukopenia and anaemia may also be seen (6).

Haematological damage may be complicated by haemorrhage of varying severity. Recurrent episodes of haemoptysis, epistaxis and severe haemorrhage requiring haemostasis procedures have been reported (6).

8. Metabolic and cardiovascular changes

Metabolic and cardiovascular alterations can also be observed, with atherogenic dyslipidaemia and increases in total cholesterol, low-density lipoprotein (LDL), and triglycerides with low HDL cholesterol (29). This leads to accelerated atherosclerosis and an increased risk of cardiovascular disease (10). Cardiac anomalies have been reported, such as valvular damage, conduction disorders or rhythm disorders such as bradycardia (16).

CHAPTER 2

ACID SPHINGOMYELINASE DEFICIENCY IN ADULTS:

WHAT ARE THE DIFFERENTIAL DIAGNOSES?

Differential diagnosis

DSMA is a rare disease with variable phenotypes, particularly in adulthood. This raises the problem of differential diagnoses, which are much more frequent in this age group. Diagnosis is mainly made with other lysosomal storage disorders, in particular Gaucher disease (30). The presence of hepatomegaly at the forefront of the diagnosis should prompt discussion of the more common liver diseases, such as chronic viral or autoimmune hepatopathy, and neoplastic causes, particularly lymphoma. Secondly, hereditary metabolic diseases should be considered, in particular overload diseases such as Gaucher's disease, lysosomal acid lipase deficiency and Niemann-Pick type C disease (30,31). The association of hepatomegaly with interstitial lung involvement should raise the suspicion of systemic disease. Systemic sarcoidosis is one of the most frequently suggested diagnoses in this context. However, the respiratory impact of sarcoidosis would be greater for the same radiological involvement. On the other hand, fibrosis in sarcoidosis is often predominant in the upper lobe. Finally, hepatomegaly and splenomegaly are much less obvious and less severe in sarcoidosis. Pulmonary fibrosis may be the main manifestation during the course of the disease. other pulmonary diseases such as idiopathic fibrosis or pulmonary alveolar proteinosis, which may include moderate hepatosplenomegaly (32).Splenomegaly is a frequent cause for investigation in internal medicine and hepato-gastrology. An exhaustive aetiological investigation is often long and laborious due to the multitude of diagnoses that can be evoked, ranging from infectious or inflammatory causes to neoplastic causes. It is therefore important to include overload diseases and hereditary metabolic diseases in decision-making algorithms.

CHAPTER 3

ACID SPHINGOMYELINASE DEFICIENCY: FROM SIMPLE INVESTIGATIONS TO DIAGNOSTIC CONFIRMATION

Initial investigations

DSMA is a rare disease with variable phenotypes. This can lead to misdiagnosis, particularly in late-onset forms. Several biological abnormalities may be observed. The presence of certain non-specific abnormalities may be of diagnostic value.

Biological check-up :

Blood count: During DSMA, certain abnormalities may be noted in the blood count, such as thrombocytopenia, leukopenia, neutropenia and anaemia (5). Lipid profile: disturbances in the lipid profile are very common in DSMA. The lipid profile is often characterised by high levels of triglycerides and total cholesterol, with low levels of HDL-cholesterol, leading to an atherogenic profile in these patients (5).

Radiological assessment:

Abdominal ultrasound: this simple examination is most often ordered as a first-line procedure when hepatomegaly and/or splenomegaly are found on physical examination. It is used to check the measurements and echogenicity of the organ explored (31). Chest X-ray: this routine examination can be used to suspect presence of interstitial lung disease (31).

CT scan: this examination is often requested to confirm the presence of interstitial lung disease and check its radiological pattern. It can also confirm the presence of organomegaly (31). Magnetic resonance imaging: this investigation is more effective in the investigation of organomegaly and in particular hepatomegaly (31). Osteo-medullary biopsy: this examination is requested in the presence of bicytopenia or pancytopenia. It reveals the presence of foamy macrophages or Niemann-Pick cells and/or sea-blue histiocytes (Figure 4). These cells are highly suggestive of the diagnosis of DSMA, but are not specific and may be observed in other lysosomal storage diseases (31).

Diagnostic confirmation :

The diagnosis is confirmed by measuring acid sphingomyelinase (SMA) activity in leukocytes or fibroblasts, the residual activity of which does not differentiate between types. Confirmation by genetic analysis is the gold standard for the diagnosis of DSMA (15).

There is a great deal of heterogeneity concerning mutations in the SMPD1 gene. Most mutations are "private" and are only found in one or a few families. Some hypotheses suggest the presence of genotype/phenotype correlations in certain cases with "common" mutations (15).

The SMPD1 ΔR610 mutation is the most frequent mutation during chronic visceral forms. This mutation is often associated with higher residual SMA activity and a less severe visceral phenotype. It is also considered to be neuroprotective whether homo or heterozygous. The A359D mutation is also associated with a predominantly visceral form with liver involvement, while the The Q294K mutation is associated with the intermediate neurovisceral phenotype NPA/B with progressive neurological impairment. The R498L, L304P and P333Sfs*52 mutations are associated with the infantile neurovisceral variant (15-17,33).

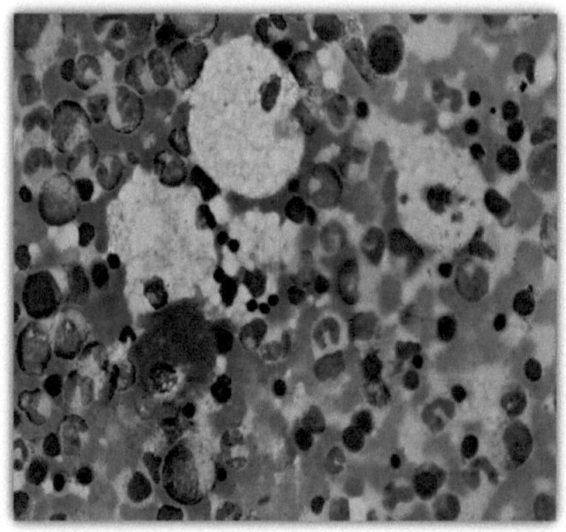

Figure 4: Myelogram showing sea-blue histiocytes after May Grünwald-Giemsa staining

CHAPTER 4

ACID SPHINGOMYELINASE DEFICIENCY: MANAGEMENT

THERAPEUTIC

Treatment

Treatment is mainly symptomatic: smoking cessation, lipid-lowering therapy and management of respiratory insufficiency. Cases of lung (34), liver (35,36) and haematopoietic stem cell (37) transplants have been reported. Olipudase alfa is an enzyme replacement therapy that treats the metabolic defect by replacing the faulty or defective SMA. To date, it is the first and only disease-modifying therapy for patents with DSMA. It currently has regulatory approval in Brazil, Japan, Europe and the United States, and is awaiting approval in other countries. (31). According to the latest recommendations published in 2023, the use of enzyme therapy should be considered in all patients with ADRD without neurological manifestations (31).

CHAPTER 5

SPHINGOMYELINASE DEFICIENCY ACID IN ADULTS:

PROGNOSIS

Prognosis

Hepatocellular failure and severe respiratory impairment are the main causes of morbidity and mortality during the course of the disease (10,18). Other causes of death have been reported, such as severe haemorrhage (of gastrointestinal origin or due to rupture of oesophageal varices, etc.) or heart failure (10,18). Cases of death from cancer have been reported in adult forms of DSMA (10,18). This highlights the importance of enzyme replacement therapy to avoid fatal outcome, as well as the importance of early detection and symptomatic treatment of organ failure.

CHAPTER 6

SPHINGOMYELINASE DEFICIENCY ACID IN ADULTS:

IMPACT ON QUALITY OF LIFE

Impact on quality of life

Studies on the impact and assessment of the quality of life of patients with hereditary metabolic diseases, and more specifically DSMA, are rare. Unlike type A, which can have major repercussions for both the patient and the family, type B appears to be a much less serious form with less psychological impact. However, the psychosocial repercussions cannot be neglected. In a study evaluating the psychosocial aspect of type B DSMA on patients and their families, a psychosocial impact was noted (38). The majority of patients evaluated reported a limitation in physical activity secondary to fatigue during the course of the disease, but also to the risks associated with certain physical activities. Patients reported that the disease had an impact on daily life. Some patients reported significant psychological repercussions, with emotional instability and an inability to fulfil their roles (38). Failure to resolve the Erikson stages was also reported in this study (38). Larger-scale studies with more exhaustive assessments seem necessary in order to better assess the impact of the disease on sufferers and to be able to provide them with psychological care.

CHAPTER 7

OUTLOOK

Outlook

MHMs, such as DSMA, present a major diagnostic challenge, particularly when they present in adulthood.

The diagnostic difficulties in this context raise significant concerns about the appropriate management of adult patients with these diseases.

As a result, the need for specialised training for adult physicians is becoming increasingly apparent. One of the main difficulties in diagnosing these conditions in adulthood is the variability and heterogeneity of the clinical manifestations.

Symptoms can be vague and non-specific, and can easily be confused with other more common conditions, delaying accurate diagnosis. In addition, MHM has long been considered a paediatric condition, leading to limited knowledge among adult physicians.

Clinicians trained primarily in adult medicine may be unfamiliar with the clinical features, biological markers and diagnostic techniques specific to these rare diseases. As a result, patients with MHMs, such as DSMA, may experience considerable diagnostic delays.

To remedy this shortcoming, it is essential to set up specific training programmes for adult doctors, focusing on MHMs. These programmes should include in-depth awareness of clinical manifestations, appropriate diagnostic approaches, management algorithms and the resources available to support patients and their families.

In addition, Interdisciplinary collaboration between medical specialists, geneticists, biochemists and allied health professionals is crucial to facilitate early and accurate diagnosis.

CONCLUSIONS

The difficulties in diagnosing MHMs, particularly when they appear in adulthood, require increased attention and specific training for adult doctors. Improving adult doctors' knowledge and awareness of these rare diseases is essential to ensure early diagnosis, appropriate management and improved quality of life for affected patients.

REFERENCES

38

1.Futerman AH, van Meer G. The cell biology of lysosomal storage disorders. Nat Rev Mol Cell Biol. 2004 Jul;5(7):554-65.

2.Futerman AH. Lysosomal diseases: pathological mechanisms and options.
therapeutics. medicine/sciences. 2005 Dec 1;21:16-9.

3.Schuchman EH, Wasserstein MP. Types A and B Niemann-Pick disease. Best Pract Res Clin Endocrinol Metab. 2015 Mar;29(2):237-47.

4.McGovern MM, Aron A, Brodie SE, Desnick RJ, Wasserstein MP. Natural history of Type A Niemann-Pick disease: possible endpoints for therapeutic trials. Neurology. 2006 Jan 24;66(2):228-32.

5.Wasserstein MP, Desnick RJ, Schuchman EH, Hossain S, Wallenstein S, Lamm C, et al. The Natural History of Type B Niemann-Pick Disease: Results From a 10- Year Longitudinal Study. Pediatrics. 2004 Dec 1;114(6):e672-7.

6.McGovern MM, Wasserstein MP, Giugliani R, Bembi B, Vanier MT, Mengel E, et al. A prospective, cross-sectional survey study of the natural history of Niemann-Pick disease type B. Pediatrics. 2008 Aug;122(2):e341-349.

7.Jezela-Stanek A, Chorostowska-Wynimko J, Tylki-Szymańska A. Pulmonary involvement in selected lysosomal storage diseases and the impact of enzyme replacement therapy: A state-of-the art review. Clin Respir J. 2020 May;14(5):422-9.

8.von Ranke FM, Pereira Freitas HM, Mançano AD, Rodrigues RS, Hochhegger B, Escuissato D, et al. Pulmonary Involvement in Niemann-Pick Disease: A State-of- the-Art Review. Lung. 2016 Aug;194(4):511-8.

9.Lidove O, Sedel F, Charlotte F, Froissart R, Vanier MT. Cirrhosis and liver failure: Expanding phenotype of acid sphingomyelinase-deficient niemann-pick disease in adulthood. JIMD Rep. 2015;15:117-21.

10. McGovern MM, Lippa N, Bagiella E, Schuchman EH, Desnick RJ, Wasserstein MP. Morbidity and mortality in type B Niemann-Pick disease. Genet Med. 2013 Aug 1;15(8):618-23.

11. Nascimbeni F, Dionisi Vici C, Vespasiani Gentilucci U,

Angelico F, Nobili V, Petta S, et al. AISF update on the diagnosis and management of adult-onset lysosomal storage diseases with hepatic involvement. Dig Liver Dis. 2020 Apr;52(4):359-67.

12. Thurberg BL, Wasserstein MP, Schiano T, O'Brien F, Richards S, Cox GF, et al. Liver and skin histopathology in adults with acid sphingomyelinase deficiency (niemann-pick disease type B). Am J Surg Pathol. 2012;36(8):1234-46.

13. Chebib N, Thivolet-Bejui F, Cottin V. Interstitial Lung Disease Associated with Adult Niemann-Pick Disease Type B. Respir Int Rev Thorac Dis. 2017;94(2):237- 8.

14. Simões RG, Maia H. Niemann-Pick type B in adulthood. BMJ Case Rep. 2015 Feb 5;2015:bcr2014208286.

15. McGovern MM, Dionisi-Vici C, Giugliani R, Hwu P, Lidove O, Lukacs Z, et al. Consensus recommendation for a diagnostic guideline for acid sphingomyelinase deficiency. Genet Med Off J Am Coll Med Genet. 2017 Sep;19(9):967-74.

16. McGovern MM, Avetisyan R, Sanson BJ, Lidove O. Disease manifestations and burden of illness in patients with acid

sphingomyelinase deficiency (ASMD). Orphanet J Rare Dis. 2017;12(1).

17. Acuña M, Martínez P, Moraga C, He X, Moraga M, Hunter B, et al. Epidemiological, clinical and biochemical characterization of the p.(Ala359Asp) SMPD1 variant causing Niemann-Pick disease type B. Eur J Hum Genet EJHG. 2016 Feb;24(2):208-13.

18. Cassiman D, Packman S, Bembi B, Turkia HB, Al-Sayed M, Schiff M, et al. Cause of death in patients with chronic visceral and chronic neurovisceral acid sphingomyelinase deficiency (Niemann-Pick disease type B and B variant): Literature review and report of new cases. Mol Genet Metab. 2016 Jul;118(3):206-13.

19. McGovern M, Wasserstein M, Bembi B, Giugliani R, Mengel E, Vanier MT, et al. Prospective study of the natural history of chronic acid sphingomyelinase deficiency in children and adults: Eleven years of observation. Mol Genet Metab. 2020 Feb;129(2):S107.

20. Sousa Martins R, Rocha S, Guimas A, Ribeiro R. Niemann-

Pick Type B: A Rare Cause of Interstitial Lung Disease. Cureus [Internet]. 2022 Jan 14 [cited 2023 Jun 24]; Available from: https://www.cureus.com/articles/79481-niemann-pick- type-b-a-rare-cause-of-interstitial-lung-disease

21. Guillemot N, Troadec C, de Villemeur TB, Clément A, Fauroux B. Lung disease in niemann-pick disease. Pediatr Pulmonol. 2007;42(12):1207-14.

22. Opoka L, Wyrostkiewicz D, Radwan-Rohrenschef P, Roży A, Tylki-Szymańska A, Tomkowski W, et al. Combined Emphysema and Interstitial Lung Disease as a Rare Presentation of Pulmonary Involvement in a Patient with Chronic Visceral Acid Sphingomyelinase Deficiency (Niemann-Pick Disease Type B). Am J Case Rep. 2020 Aug 6;21:e923394.

23. Gülhan B, Özçelik U, Gürakan F, Güçer Ş, Orhan D, Cinel G, et al. Different features of lung involvement in Niemann-Pick disease and Gaucher disease. Respir Med. 2012 Sep 1;106(9):1278-85.

24. Imaging Manifestations of Niemann-Pick Disease Type B | AJR [Internet]. [cited 2023 Jul 3]. Available from:

https://www.ajronline.org/doi/10.2214/AJR.09.2871

25. Ahuja J, Kanne JP, Meyer CA, Pipavath SNJ, Schmidt RA, Swanson JO, et al. Histiocytic Disorders of the Chest: Imaging Findings. RadioGraphics [Internet]. 2015 Mar 12 [cited 2023 Jul 3]; Available from: https://pubs.rsna.org/doi/10.1148/rg.352140197

26. Alizon C, Beucher AB, Gourdier AL, Lavigne C. Niemann-Pick type B disease: clinical description of three familial cases. Rev Médecine Interne. 2010 Aug;31(8):562-5.

27. Wasserstein M, Godbold J, McGovern MM. Skeletal manifestations in pediatric and adult patients with Niemann Pick disease type B. J Inherit Metab Dis. 2013;36(1):123-7.

28. Arenz C. Small Molecule Inhibitors of Acid Sphingomyelinase. Cell Physiol Biochem. 2010;26(1):1-8.

29. McGovern MM, Pohl-Worgall T, Deckelbaum RJ, Simpson W, Mendelson D, Desnick RJ, et al. Lipid abnormalities in children with types A and B Niemann Pick disease. J Pediatr. 2004 Jul 1;145(1):77-81.

30. Cappellini MD, Motta I, Barbato A, Giuffrida G, Manna R,

Carubbi F, et al. Similarities and differences between Gaucher disease and acid sphingomyelinase deficiency: An algorithm to support the diagnosis. Eur J Intern Med. 2023 Feb;108:81-4.

31. Geberhiwot T, Wasserstein M, Wanninayake S, Bolton SC, Dardis A, Lehman A, et al. Consensus clinical management guidelines for acid sphingomyelinase deficiency (Niemann-Pick disease types A, B and A/B). Orphanet J Rare Dis. 2023;18(1).

32. Jouneau S, Kerjouan M, Briens E, Lenormand JP, Meunier C, Letheulle J, et al. Pulmonary alveolar proteinosis. Rev Mal Respir. 2014 Dec 1;31(10):975-91.

33. Simonaro CM, Desnick RJ, McGovern MM, Wasserstein MP, Schuchman EH. The Demographics and Distribution of Type B Niemann-Pick Disease: Novel Mutations Lead to New Genotype/Phenotype Correlations. Am J Hum Genet. 2002 Dec 1;71(6):1413-9.

34. Mannem H, Kilbourne S, Weder M. Lung transplantation in a patient with Niemann-Pick disease. J Heart Lung Transplant. 2019 Jan;38(1):100-1.

35. Coelho GR, Praciano AM, Rodrigues JPC, Viana CFG,

Brandão KP, Valenca JTJ, et al. Liver Transplantation in Patients With Niemann-Pick Disease--Single-Center Experience. Transplant Proc. 2015 Dec;47(10):2929-31.

36. Liu Y, Luo Y, Xia L, Qiu B, Zhou T, Feng M, et al. The Effects of Liver Transplantation in Children With Niemann-Pick Disease Type B. Liver Transplant Off Publ Am Assoc Study Liver Dis Int Liver Transplant Soc. 2019 Aug;25(8):1233-40.

37. Quarello P, Spada M, Porta F, Vassallo E, Timeus F, Fagioli F. Hematopoietic stem cell transplantation in Niemann-Pick disease type B monitored by chitotriosidase activity. Pediatr Blood Cancer. 2018 Feb;65(2).

38. Henderson SL, Packman W, Packman S. Psychosocial aspects of patients with Niemann-Pick disease, type B. Am J Med Genet A. 2009 Nov;149A(11):2430-6.

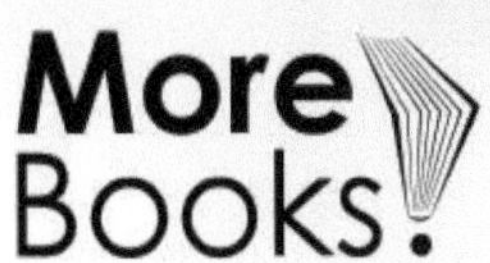

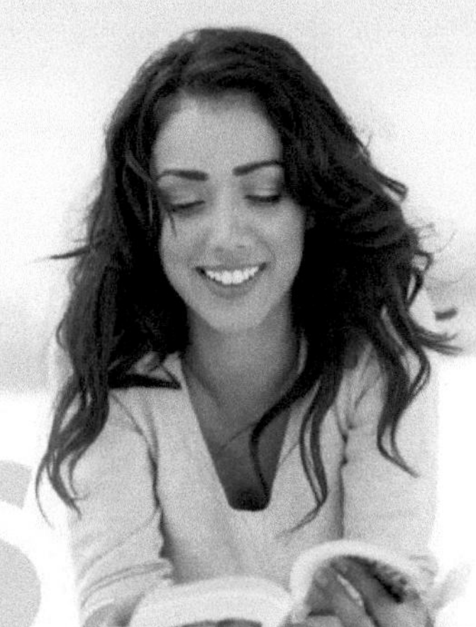

yes I want morebooks!

Buy your books fast and straightforward online - at one of world's fastest growing online book stores! Environmentally sound due to Print-on-Demand technologies.

Buy your books online at
www.morebooks.shop

Kaufen Sie Ihre Bücher schnell und unkompliziert online – auf einer der am schnellsten wachsenden Buchhandelsplattformen weltweit! Dank Print-On-Demand umwelt- und ressourcenschonend produziert.

Bücher schneller online kaufen
www.morebooks.shop

info@omniscriptum.com
www.omniscriptum.com

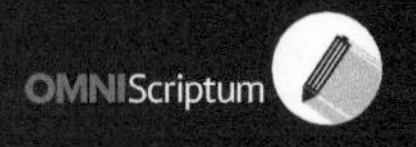

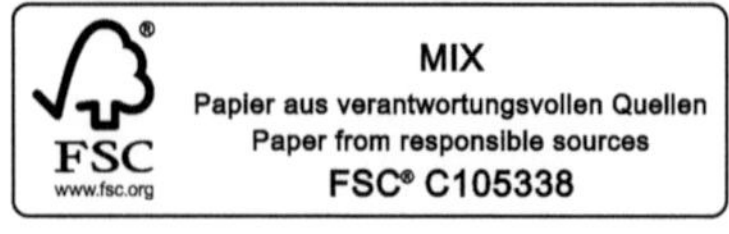

Printed by Books on Demand GmbH, Norderstedt / Germany